the little book of
CHAKRAS

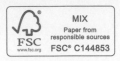

First published in 2022 by OH!
An Imprint of Welbeck Non-Fiction Limited,
part of Welbeck Publishing Group.
Based in London and Sydney.
www.welbeckpublishing.com

Disclaimer:
This book is intended for general informational purposes only and should not be relied upon as recommending or promoting any specific practice, diet or method of treatment. It is not intended to diagnose, advise, treat or prevent any illness or condition and is not a substitute for advice from a professional practitioner of the subject matter contained in this book. You should not use the information in this book as a substitute for medication, nutritional, diet, spiritual or other treatment that is prescribed by your practitioner. The publisher makes no representations or warranties with respect to the accuracy, completeness or currency of the contents of this work, and specifically disclaim, without limitation, any implied warranties of merchantability or fitness for a particular purpose and any injury, illness, damage, death, liability or loss incurred, directly or indirectly from the use or application of any of the contents of this book. Furthermore, the publisher is not affiliated with and does not sponsor or endorse any uses of or beliefs about in any way referred in this book.

ISBN 978-1-80069-178-0

Compiled and written by: Lisa Dyer
Editorial: Victoria Godden
Project manager: Russell Porter
Design: Andy Jones
Production: Jess Brisley

A CIP catalogue record for this book is available from the British Library

Printed in China

10 9 8 7 6 5 4 3 2 1

Illustrations: Freepik.com

the little book of
CHAKRAS

lisa dyer

CONTENTS

INTRODUCTION

In this beginner's introduction to chakra energy work, you will learn all about the seven main chakras, as well as many other energy centres, how to identify if they are out of balance and how to activate and align them to encourage flow and vitality throughout the body.

Basic information on chakras and chakra healing, including an overview of the different systems, is covered in the first chapter. The lower and upper chakra chapters discuss the seven main chakras in detail, including their associations with elements, planets, colours and body systems as well as crystals, herbs and essential oils to use in chakra-balancing practices. Here you will also discover how to identify if a particular chakra is unbalanced, overactive, underactive or blocked. The fourth chapter discusses the secondary and minor chakras, other energy points and channels of the body.

Various ways to use meditation, visualization, affirmations, breathing and yoga poses to activate and balance specific chakras are given in the fifth chapter, while the use of crystals, herbs and essential oils are explored in rituals and practices in the sixth chapter.

When working with your chakras, the aim is balance, so avoid focusing too much on one chakra over another. The whole point is to identify where you need help on a day-to-day basis and realign holistically. One day your lower chakras may all be well balanced, but your heart or throat chakra is underactive, leading to a stagnation of the upper chakras – and spiritual disconnection. Or you may find that your solar plexus is underactive and you're suffering from low confidence and digestive problems. Learning about each chakra and checking in with them each day will help ensure excellent flow of energy and nourish your physical, emotional and spiritual health.

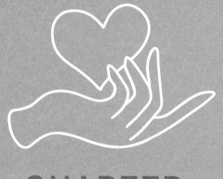

CHAPTER

1

the ENERGY CONNECTION

Discover the energy system
of the chakras, their traditional and
cultural origins, and the basics of
chakra healing.

WHAT are
CHAKRAS?

A holistic energy system,
the chakras are focal points in
the body where energetic
forces and bodily functions
connect and interact with each
other, affecting emotional,
spiritual and physical wellbeing.

Many consider the chakras as doorways or gates to perception.

If they are open and aligned, they are balanced, but any one or several of them can be blocked or out of alignment at any time.

The seven primary chakras are the ones most discussed, however there are five secondaries, as well as minor chakras and other energetic centres.

The total number within the body (and in the dimensions and aura around the human body) varies widely according to different traditions; common systems are based on 5, 7, 12, 21 or 114 chakras.

"Each of the seven chakras are governed by spiritual laws, principles of consciousness that we can use to cultivate greater harmony, happiness and wellbeing in our lives and in the world."

Deepak Chopra

Chakras were first recorded in India between 1500 and 500 BCE in the Vedas, where they were mentioned as "cakras".

In Buddhism and Jainism, chakra means "wheel" or the "wheel of dharma", and the chakras can be envisioned as spinning wheels or vortexes of free-flowing positive energy in the body.

The seven-chakra system commonly used today was first seen in the *Kubjikāmata-Tantra*, an eleventh-century Shaivism/Shaktism religious text, which was translated by Sir John Woodroffe in the early twentieth century.

the seven main chakras

The chakra energy points start at the root, or base, of the spine and extend to the crown of the head, and opening up these chakras from root to crown reflects the journey of spiritual ascent *(see chapters 2 and 3 for detailed information on each one).*

1 **the root chakra**

2 **the sacral chakra**

3 **the solar plexus chakra**

4 **the heart chakra**

5 **the throat chakra**

6 **the third eye chakra**

7 **the crown chakra**

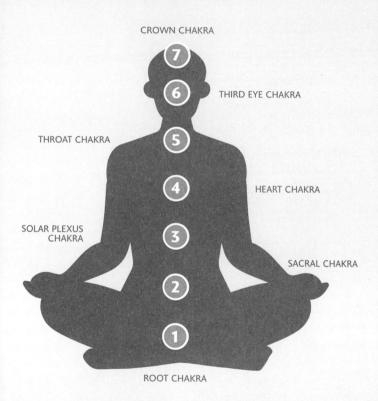

CROWN CHAKRA

THIRD EYE CHAKRA

THROAT CHAKRA

HEART CHAKRA

SOLAR PLEXUS
CHAKRA

SACRAL CHAKRA

ROOT CHAKRA

what do the chakras do?

The function depends on the chakra, however when all are balanced, open and aligned, you will feel a sense of harmony in all areas of your life.

When a chakra is out of balance, this indicates the specific energy that is lacking or where you need to focus attention or grow. Your actions and emotions also affect the chakras; for example, if you are experiencing grief or heartbreak, your heart chakra may close or become inactive.

Here are a few of the general uses of chakra balancing and healing.

- Heal physical illnesses
- Clear stagnant energy
- Release emotional blocks
- Stimulate flow of energy throughout the body, increasing vitality
- Increase focus and concentration
- Improve confidence and self-control
- Stabilize mood
- Encourage a positive outlook
- Heighten creativity and perception
- Increase psychic powers

secondary and minor chakras

Work in quantum physics and energy healing has aided the exploration of many other energy vortexes, though there are various schools of thought on the number and their correspondences to the primary chakras.

There are thought to be 114 chakras in total in the body, and by mastering the powers of the minor chakras you can master the primary ones too.

"*We have five senses in which we glory and which we recognize and celebrate, senses that constitute the sensible world for us. But there are other senses – secret senses, sixth senses, if you will – equally vital, but unrecognized, and unlauded.*"

Oliver Sacks,
The Man Who Mistook His Wife for a Hat (1985)

yin and yang energies

The chakra system integrates both feminine (yin) and masculine (yang) energies, and each chakra is associated with one or a particular balance of both. Yin and yang are two different halves that when united form a perfect wholeness; they are opposing but interdependent. In chakra work, it is useful to consider whether you are having blockages in the chakras associated with yin or yang, as this can help you to rebalance.

Yin qualities: spirituality, coolness, moistness, night, winter, earth, rest

Yang qualities: physicality, warmth, dryness, day, summer, space, activity

the kundalini connection

In Hinduism, kundalini, or "coiled power", is a divine feminine energy residing in the base of the spine and identified as a snake rising upwards through the chakras, through the central meridian (*nadi*), achieving different layers of experience until it reaches profound spiritual transformation at the crown.

Kundalini is said to awaken in earth with the sense of smell in the root chakra; take in water and taste in the sacral chakra; ignite fire and form in the solar plexus; take in air and touch in the throat; ether and sound in the third eye; and finally transforming into the white moon.

balanced and unbalanced chakras

When all seven chakras are aligned, balanced and open, there is a stable, constant flow of energy through the body. You feel at one mentally, emotionally, physically and spiritually.

Chakras become unbalanced when they are overactive or underactive, blocked or closed.

Here are some ways to identify a general imbalance.

- General sense of being off-kilter or out-of-sync
- Feeling sluggish, lethargic and unmotivated
- Alternatively, feeling hyper, nervous, tense and high-strung
- Life feels chaotic and unsettled
- Experiencing doubt or insecurities about your direction in life
- Inability to make decisions
- Low confidence and self-esteem
- Depression or mood swings
- Physical ailments, such as stiffness, aches and pains, and headaches

overactive and underactive chakras

A chakra is described as being overactive if it is creating excess energy and working too hard, or if it is compensating for a lack elsewhere.

An underactive chakra is not a closed chakra, but just an underperformer! It's not functioning at a high enough level or vibration, and needs rebalancing to come back to a healthy state. Notice too if a chakra feels like it is losing too much energy or holding on to too much energy.

closed or blocked energy

When any one chakra becomes blocked
or completely closed, it can not only
cause the dysfunction of that chakra but
also disrupt the flow of energy throughout
the entire body.

chakra healing

The mind–body connection of chakra healing is especially potent for curing physical ailments.

As each chakra is associated with an organ and bodily function (for example, the root with the adrenal glands), clearing and strengthening that chakra can alleviate problems associated with that specific part of the body.

"Disease is often an accumulation of dammed-up energy. When we learn how energy moves through the chakras we can begin to allow it to flow freely through our bodies, creating greater health."

Caroline Shola Arewa,
The Way of the Chakras (2012)

SIGNS AND SYMBOLS

Early Sanskrit texts speak of chakras as meditative visualizations combining flowers and mantras and as physical entities in the body.

Each of the chakras is symbolized by a lotus flower bud with a specified number of petals. As each petal opens, various experiences and awakenings take place, culminating with the opening of that chakra.

Here are some of the symbols you will see associated with the chakras.

circle: The chakra "wheel", infinity, unity and the cyclical nature of energy.

inverted triangle: The alchemical symbol for earth.

six-pointed star: Consisting of two triangles, this represents the yin and yang.

crescent moon: A connection with creativity and the feminine.

WORKING WITH THE CHAKRAS

There are many ways to activate, balance and heal your chakras – many of these are used in the projects in chapters 5 and 6.

Use them alone or combine them (for example, crystals with meditation; yoga with essential oils and colour therapy) for extra potency.

Note: When using essential oils in any topical applications, always do a patch test beforehand to ensure you do not have any sensitivity.

candles: Choose candles in colours and scents associated with the chakra you are working with, and use them in your home, on an altar or in your meditative practice.

colour: Enhance the power of the chakra by wearing the colour associated with that chakra, in scarves, clothing or jewellery; in home furnishings; or eat fresh fruits and vegetables in those colours.

crystals: These can be worn, carried in a pocket, used to charge drinks or baths, placed on altars or formed on grids. Clear quartz is the amplifier, so although not associated with a particular chakra, it will enhance the energy of the other stones you use.

Essential oils: These can be used in diffusers for fragrance, inhaled, applied directly to the skin when diluted in a carrier oil or added to a body treatment or bath.

Flowers, herbs and roots: Use the herb, flower or spice associated with the chakra you are balancing in food, teas and infusions, or add them to a bath. You may also like to meditate on a specific flower, herb or plant, indoors or outside in a garden or park.

Mantras and affirmations: Sound connects the mind and body and is a wonderful way to enhance your chakra balancing as well as your breathwork. Use a tone that is natural and comfortable for the duration of a breath, then keep repeating.

Meditations and visualizations: Excellent for focusing on and opening up the chakras, a standard practice involves working through all chakras from the root to the crown, visualizing them as spinning wheels or opening lotus blooms in their associated colours. Start by concentrating on the lower chakras to create a strong foundation before moving on to higher-chakra work.

Mudras: Each chakra is associated with a different hand gesture, and using these in meditation and visualization practice, especially when combined with the relevant mantra, can enhance the connection to your energy centre.

Sound: Gongs, tuning forks and singing bowls can all be used to increase the vibrational frequency of chakras. The chakras correspond to particular notes: use C for the root chakra; D for sacral; E for solar plexus; F for heart; G for throat; A for the third eye; and B for the crown.

Toning or humming: Use your own voice to activate a chakra by placing both hands on the chakra that needs balancing, then begin to hum deeply, gradually getting higher in pitch. When you begin to feel the chakra responding to that tone, use that pitch for as long as you are able. Repeat daily.

Yoga: Specific yoga poses are excellent for different chakras; for example, sitting asanas are great for the root chakra, while neck and shoulder openers, such as the Camel and Cat-Cow, are best for opening up the throat chakra.

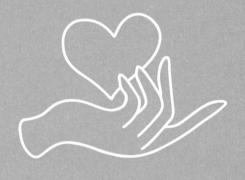

CHAPTER

2

the LOWER CHAKRAS

Learn in-depth information on the root, sacral and solar plexus chakras, their locations, attributes and associations, and how to tell when they are out of balance.

THE PHYSICAL BODY

The lower chakras rule over the physical body, your relationship to the physical world and your emotional identity. They keep you grounded and stable and connect to the upper chakras via the heart chakra.

"Walk as if you are kissing the Earth with your feet."

Thich Nhat Hanh,
Peace Is Every Step (1990)

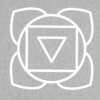

1: ROOT CHAKRA

Also called the base chakra, this chakra governs basic needs, security, trust and aspects of the physical body. The root chakra receives energy from the earth and is concerned with the fundamental requirements of life – food, shelter, clothing and money.

Sanskrit name: *Muladhara*

Mula means "root" and *adhara* means "support" or "base", and the word can be interpreted as "the root of existence".

Key Affirmation: I am.

Key attributes: Security, safety, survival, stability

Colour: Red

Symbol: Four-petalled lotus flower with an inverted triangle

Mantra: "Lam"

Location: Base of the spine

Element: Earth

Planets: Earth and Saturn

Energy: Masculine

Animal: Elephant

Day: Saturday

Zodiac signs: Taurus and Virgo

Body systems: Bones and adrenal glands

Herbs and essential oils: Ashwagandha, black pepper, cedarwood, dandelion root, frankincense, hibiscus, myrrh, patchouli, raspberry leaf, sandalwood, vetiver

Crystals: Black tourmaline, garnet, hematite, red jasper, smoky quartz

Balanced: You feel grounded, safe and connected, and your energy is strong and stable.

Unbalanced: You feel uncertain, fearful and anxious, low in energy, and you may become greedy or paranoid.

WORK WITH THE ROOT CHAKRA FOR:

Grounding and being present in the body

Body-image disorders

Childhood trauma or instability

Family or home issues

Stress and the fight-or-flight response

Confidence and feeling more centred –
particularly if you feel you are being
swayed too much by others

2: SACRAL CHAKRA

The centre of emotions, relationships, sexuality and creativity, the sacral chakra is also concerned with flow, flexibility and fun. Essential for a positive attitude to, and enjoyment of, life, the chakra radiates warmth and vitality. It is connected to our relationships with our self and others.

Sanskrit name: *Svadhisthana*

   Swa means "self" and *adhishthana*
   means "abode" or "seat", and the
   word can be interpreted as "the
   dwelling place of the self".

Key Affirmation: I Feel.

Key attributes: Passion, creativity, emotion, desire, pleasure

Colour: Orange

Symbol: Circle with six-petalled flower with a crescent moon

Mantra: "Vam"

Location: Lower abdomen, between the pelvis and navel

Element: Water

Planets: Jupiter and the Moon

Energy: Feminine

Animal: Crocodile

Days: Monday, Thursday and Friday

Zodiac signs: Scorpio and Leo

Body systems: Lymphatic system; ovaries and testicles

Herbs and essential oils: Bergamot, calendula, fennel, ginseng, mandarin, nasturtium, neroli, orange, ylang ylang

Crystals: Carnelian, orange calcite, sunstone, moonstone

Balanced: You feel creative, desirable and full of possibility and abundance.

Unbalanced: You may feel disconnected, uninspired, shameful about sex or your sexuality, and exhibit co-dependency, hedonistic behaviour or addictions.

WORK WITH THE SACRAL CHAKRA FOR:

Guilt

Apathy

Creative stagnancy

Repression of emotions or desires

Menstruation or fertility issues

High emotional states and difficulty
    controlling the emotions

Addictions or bad habits

"True creativity often starts where language ends."

Arthur Koestler,
The Act of Creation (1964)

"*Pleasure is the sun of the morning, the cloud of the meridian, and the storm of the evening.*"

William Scott Downey,
Proverbs (2016)

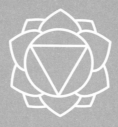

3: SOLAR PLEXUS CHAKRA

Associated with wisdom, personal power, self-esteem and transformation, this chakra is concerned with who we really are and our purpose. It is believed to have a magnetic effect that attracts energy from the universe to the self and promotes a fiery "warrior" energy.

Sanskrit name: *Manipura*

Mani, meaning "gem", and *pura*, meaning "city", makes the literal translation "the city of jewels", often interpreted as being your central powerhouse of gifts and talents.

Key Affirmation: I Do.

Key attributes: Confidence, willpower, joy, success, momentum

Colour: Yellow

Symbol: A ten-petalled circle with an inverted triangle

Mantra: "Ram"

Location: Upper abdomen

Element: Fire

Planet: Mars

Energy: Masculine

Animal: Ram

Day: Tuesday

Zodiac signs: Aries and Sagittarius

Body systems: Digestive system, and liver, spleen, gallbladder and pancreas

Herbs and essential oils: Chamomile, ginger, lemon, lemongrass, rosemary, turmeric

Crystals: Citrine, yellow tourmaline, tiger's eye, pyrite

Balanced: You feel motivated, confident, self-disciplined, self-sufficient and independent.

Unbalanced: You suffer from low self-esteem, neediness, lack of direction or motivation, or the opposite: control-freakiness and manipulation.

WORK WITH THE SOLAR PLEXUS CHAKRA FOR:

Greater motivation and willpower

Decision-making

Achieving goals

Stomach problems and weight gain

Fatigue

"I will not die an unlived life ... I choose to inhabit my days, to allow my living to open me, to make me less afraid, more accessible, to loosen my heart until it becomes a wing, a torch, a promise.

Dawna Markova,
I Will Not Die an Unlived Life (2010)

"In the chakra system, the solar plexus is the seat of personal power. Power is not about exerting our will over others; it is about being in complete truth with yourself."

Madisyn Taylor,
co-founder of DailyOM.com

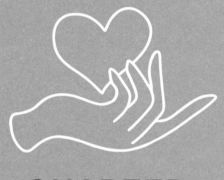

CHAPTER

3

the UPPER CHAKRAS

Discover the locations, attributes and associations of the heart chakra, which bridges the lower and upper chakras as well as the throat, third eye and crown chakras.

THE SPIRITUAL SELF

The higher chakras rule over your more spiritual self, connecting you to the universal and enlightenment. These chakras will help you manifest your best self and feel a connection with the universe and divine love.

"From within or from behind, a light shines through us upon things and makes us aware that we are nothing, but the light is all."

Ralph Waldo Emerson,
Self-Reliance, the Over-Soul and Other Essays (2010)

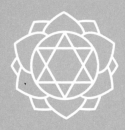

4: HEART CHAKRA

Bridging the earthly and spiritual, the lower and higher chakras, the heart chakra promotes love, serenity, balance and healing. It is responsible for compassion, unconditional love and transcending judgement and black-and-white thinking.

Sanskrit name: *Anahata*

Translating as "unhurt" or "unbeaten'" in Sanskrit, the fourth chakra is often interpreted to mean the ability to hear the celestial world, the "unstruck sound".

Key Affirmation: I Love.

Key attributes: Love, compassion, empathy, forgiveness, relationships, beauty in life

Colours: Pink and green

Symbol: Two intersecting triangles forming a six-pointed star in a circle with 12 petals

Mantra: "Yam"

Location: Centre of the chest

Element: Air

Planet: Venus

Energy: Feminine

Animals: Antelope and dove

Days: Wednesday and Friday

Zodiac sign: Cancer

Body systems: Cardiac and lungs; vagus nerve and thymus

Herbs and essential oils: Geranium, honeysuckle, hyssop, jasmine, rose, rosehip

Crystals: Emerald, green aventurine, jade, rhodochrosite, rose quartz

Balanced: You feel trusting, affectionate and forgiving, and maintain meaningful relationships.

Unbalanced: You may feel isolated, defensive, victimized or are suffering from overwhelming grief or sadness.

WORK WITH THE HEART CHAKRA FOR:

Self-criticism

Forgiveness of yourself or others

Loneliness and grief

Romance and heartbreak

Relationship issues, particularly
imbalanced ones

Repressed emotions or a closed heart

Heart arrhythmias or murmurs, blood
pressure problems

"You yourself, as much as anybody in the entire universe, deserve your love and affection."

Buddha

"*Peace is this moment without judgement,*

this moment in the Heart-space where

everything that is, is welcome."

Dorothy Hunt,
"Peace Is This Moment Without Judgement"

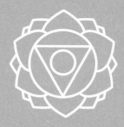

5: THROAT CHAKRA

Strongly connected to communication and the ability to connect with your truth and share it, the throat chakra is associated with the spirit and higher consciousness. It is often seen as a "bottleneck" of energy flow in the body due to its location.

Sanskrit name: *Vishuddha*

From *shuddhi*, meaning "pure", and
vi, which intensifies *shuddhi*, the
translation is "especially pure" and
connects to honesty and truth. In
teachings, the body is thought to
have reached a purified state if this
chakra is in balance.

Key Affirmation: I Speak.

Key attributes: Communication, truth, expression, authenticity, good timing

Colour: Turquoise

Symbol: An inverted triangle inside a circle with 16 petals

Mantra: "Ham"

Location: Throat

Element: Ether

Planets: Mercury and Jupiter

Energy: Masculine

Animal: Lion

Day: Thursday

Zodiac signs: Gemini and Aquarius

Body systems: Thyroid, which regulates processing energy through temperature and metabolism; also the mouth, throat, jaws, palate and the shoulders and neck

Herbs and essential oils: Basil, eucalyptus, geranium, peppermint, sage, tea tree

Crystals: Amazonite, angelite, aquamarine, hemimorphite, larimar

Balanced: You speak confidently and truthfully, realize your purpose and possess strong willpower.

Unbalanced: You may have difficulty expressing your feelings and thoughts or suffer from stumbling over words, poor listening skills, talking over others or interrupting, and social anxiety; at worst, you may engage in secretiveness, gossiping and lying.

WORK WITH THE THROAT CHAKRA FOR:

Public speaking

Social anxiety and nervousness

Better two-way communication

Active listening

Expression of thoughts

Amplifying your voice or message

Sore throats or laryngitis

"*The universe is full of magical things, patiently waiting for our wits to grow sharper.*"

Eden Phillpotts,
A Shadow Passes (1919)

"The immortal part of man shakes off from itself, one after the other, its outer casings and – as the snake from its skin, the butterfly from its chrysalis – emerges from one after another, passing into a higher state of consciousness."

Annie Besant,
Theosophical Review (1892)

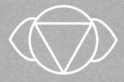

6: THIRD EYE OR BROW CHAKRA

Connecting to intuition, awareness, intelligence, and vision, this chakra transcends time and is primarily concerned with perception – the ability to see both inner and outer worlds, and receive messages about the past or future. The point of view is objective, transcending self-limiting beliefs and dualities of black and white or good and bad.

Sanskrit name: *Ajna*

Meaning "perceive", "command"
or "beyond wisdom", it is said to
be the "eye of consciousness", the
point at which spiritual energy from
nature enters the body, giving the
gift of seeing the world clearly.

Key Affirmation: I See.

Key attributes: Insight, perception, intuition, intellect

Colour: Indigo or purple

Symbol: An inverted triangle between two lotus petals

Mantra: "Aum"

Location: Between the eyebrows

Element: Light

Planets: Jupiter and Venus

Energy: Feminine

Animal: Hawk

Days: Thursday and Friday

Zodiac signs: Libra and Pisces

Body systems: Pineal gland (in charge of regulating biorhythms, including sleep and waking times), the brain and eyes

Herbs and essential oils: Blue lotus, eyebright, jasmine, mugwort, passionflower

Crystals: Azurite, blue kyanite, labradorite, lapis lazuli, sodalite

Balanced: You have a strong sense of intuition, energy perception and are spiritual

Unbalanced: You may feel confused, erratic, find it difficult to read a room or see the big picture. You may also feel stuck, misanthropic or arrogant.

WORK WITH THE THIRD EYE CHAKRA FOR:

Decision-making and clarity

Greater concentration and focus

Imagination

Perception and psychic abilities

Headaches and eye problems

Insomnia

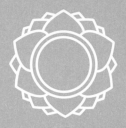

7: CROWN CHAKRA

Known as the "bridge to the Cosmos",
the crown chakra focuses on the
knowledge and understanding that is
beyond what words can describe – the
universal consciousness. Spirituality
and higher consciousness are the
hallmarks of this uppermost chakra.

Sanskrit name: *Sahasrara*

Meaning "thousand petalled", the Sanskrit word denotes the divine lotus or the "seat of God", and signifies the attainment of liberation for the enlightened.

Key Affirmation: I Know.

Key attributes: Spirituality, enlightenment, wisdom, higher consciousness

Colour: Violet or white

Symbol: Concentric rings of flower petals

Mantra: Silence

Location: Top of the head – or four finger-widths above

Element: Cosmos

Planets: Sun and Uranus

Energy: Masculine and feminine

Animal: Eagle

Zodiac sign: Capricorn

Day: Sunday

Body systems: Pituitary gland primarily, brain and nervous system; pineal and hypothalamus

Herbs and essential oils: Gotu kola, holy basil, lavender, pink lotus

Crystals: Amethyst, clear quartz, moonstone, selenite

Balanced: You enjoy feelings of peace, spiritual fulfilment, being at one with the universe and transcendence.

Unbalanced: You may feel fearful, lacking in belief or depressed; at worst, you may exhibit selfishness, high-handedness and live too much in the head.

WORK WITH THE CROWN CHAKRA FOR:

Disillusionment

Depression

Lack of purpose or belief

Self-obsession and ego

Too much focus on the past or future

Greater self-awareness

Spiritual growth and enlightenment

CHAPTER

4

SECONDARY
and MINOR
CHAKRAS

Learn about the additional five energy vortexes – the earth star, lunar, solar, galactic, universal energy vortexes outside the body, as well as other minor chakras and nadis within the body.

the 12 and 21 systems

With the 12-chakra system, there are two main schools of thought regarding the additional five chakras, often termed the "secondary" chakras.

The first characterizes a chakra that lies in the earth with an additional four above the crown, which is the system shown here. The alternative system relates to five additional chakras that are located in between the seven primaries.

The minor chakras, of which there are up to 114 (which some practitioners refer to as energy points rather than chakras, as they reside within the body) are usually agreed to form a core of 21.

"You are the universe expressing itself as a human for a little while."

Eckhart Tolle

8: EARTH STAR CHAKRA

Located below the root chakra, this chakra is sometimes labelled as number "0" on chakra charts. It is often called the "super root" as it is deeper than the root chakra and is the anchor for the whole system. It penetrates into the earth and its underground, connecting to the magnetic core of the earth.

Key attributes: Deep grounding and stability; fosters connection with the planet and the environment; helps to stay present in the here and now; life-nurturing.

Colour: Brown

Location: 12–18 inches (30–45 cm) below the feet

Crystals: Flint, red jasper, tiger's eye

WORK WITH THE EARTH STAR CHAKRA FOR:

Deep grounding and earth connection

Strong physical health

Past choices and applying past knowledge to the present

Ancestry and past lives

Balancing those who are very spiritual or suffer from dizziness

"*Surely a man needs a closed place wherein he may strike root and, like the seed, become. But also he needs the great Milky Way above him and the vast sea spaces, though neither stars nor ocean serve his daily needs.*"

Antoine de Saint-Exupéry,
The Wisdom of the Sands (1948)

9: LUNAR CHAKRA

Located above the head, directly above the seventh crown chakra, it connects with the power of the moon, the divine feminine and enlightenment. It is good for karmic therapy, emotional healing and connecting with spiritual guides and the angelic realm.

Key attributes: Feminine energy,
emotions and spirituality

Colours: Silver and white

Location: 6 inches (15 cm) above the
crown chakra

Crystals: Moonstone and white
selenite

10: SOLAR CHAKRA

This chakra contains the energy of light itself. It is associated with the sun, masculine energy, purification and illumination. Combine the practice with the lunar chakra to harness the forces of both female and masculine energy.

Key attributes: Masculine energy, vitality and creative powers

Colour: Gold

Location: Above the lunar chakra

Crystals: Citrine and yellow topaz

11: GALACTIC CHAKRA

This is a strong healing chakra that connects with the solar plexus to dissolve ego and heal emotional trauma, especially from your past. It can also help you explore past lives.

Key attributes: Healing and advanced spiritual skills

Colours: Violet with gold and silver

Location: Above the solar chakra

Crystals: Ametrine or amethyst and citrine used together

12: UNIVERSAL CHAKRA

Located above all the chakras and the body's aura, this chakra is known as the energy of universal unity and togetherness. It is associated with the deepest meditation and the collective unconscious, and it enhances the crown chakra.

Key attributes: Transformational energy, cosmic travel

Colour: Iridescence

Location: Above the galactic chakra

Crystal: Rainbow topaz

THE 21 MINOR CHAKRAS

Sometimes called the energy centres, these are powerful but small energy acupoints that are "reflected points" of the seven major chakras, having similar properties to their counterparts and dealing with body functions.

There are many minor chakras distributed all over the body, which are created by criss-crossing energy lines, but most teachings refer to those described here. Like the primary chakras, they can also have emotional and energetic blockages.

Ear points: 2
With one in front of each ear close to the jawbone, these relate to the hearing and understanding of guidance, knowledge and providing a balanced perspective. They are associated with the heart chakra.

Eyes: 2
With one behind each eye, they relate to clear seeing, sixth sense and intuition, and are associated with the third eye chakra.

Elbows: 2
Located in each of the inner elbows, these relate to your ability to stand your ground and argue your points and are associated with the root chakra.

Knees: 2

With one on the back of each knee,
these are linked to your physical flexibility
and to your attitude and ability to adapt.
Working with the knees can help you
with fears related to death and change.
These chakras are ssociated with the
root chakra.

Hands: 2

Located in the palm of each hand, these
are associated with the flow of life energy
and are symbolic of giving and receiving,
as well as healing. They are associated
with the heart and crown chakras.

Feet: 2

Located in the sole of each foot, these
are linked to all the organs of the body, as
in the practice of reflexology, as well
as stability and endurance. They are
associated with the root chakra.

Breast: 2

With one above each breast, these are
linked to physical needs, such as nutrition,
as well as emotional needs. They are
associated with the heart chakra.

Clavicle: 2

Located above the breast chakras at the
clavicle, these are linked to respiration,
lungs and breath. They are associated with
the throat chakra.

Thymus: 1
Located below the throat chakra, midway
between the heart and the throat, where
the thymus intersects the Vagus nerve,
this corresponds to self-esteem and
inner peace and the immune system. It is
associated with the heart chakra.

Spleen: 1
Some sources consider this chakra as two
superimposed energy points. Either way,
it is located at the spleen and helps with
toxins as well as releasing negativity and
eliminating destructive behaviour and
bad habits. It is associated with the solar
plexus chakra.

Liver: 1
Found in the area of your liver, this chakra helps with detoxification and boosts digestion, and is associated with the solar plexus chakra.

Ovaries/Gonads: 2
Located in the groin, these are linked to fertility and sexuality, and are associated with the sacral chakra in women and the root chakra in men.

THE ALTA MAJOR CHAKRA

Also known as the "Mouth of the Goddess", the "Well of Dreams" and the Zeal point, and sometimes referred to as the back of the third eye chakra, this vortex is located at the back of the neck.

It is acknowledged to be one of the most important minor chakras and is best for those already established in their chakra practice. It is associated with the atlas bone – the first vertebrae of the spine, where the cranial bones connect with the spine.

Key attributes: Stores past life knowledge, connects to divine inspiration, clarity of mind and purpose, fresh perspectives

Colour: Teal blue

Location: Nape of the neck

Herbs and essential oils: Juniper, sandalwood, star anise, vetiver

Crystals: Black touramaline, angelinite, aurichalcite, afghanite, blue kyanite or blue moonstone

Balanced: A gateway to access higher dimensions and expand awareness; refreshes energy.

Unbalanced: You may suffer from tinnitus or pressure in the ears, dizziness, headaches and sinus problems, a stiff neck and painful jaw. It can also be an entry point for psychic attacks.

TO WORK WITH THE ALTA MAJOR CHAKRA:

Protect it with a scarf tied around the neck

Guard the back of your neck with an
upturned collar

Anoint the area with essential oils or sprays

Feed it with high vibrations, such as with
craniosacral therapy

OTHER HIGHER MINOR CHAKRAS

Forehead chakra: On the fontanel, this deals with the thalamus and is linked to the third eye.

Chandra chakra: Between the third eye and the crown, this is associated with the moon and deals with forgiveness and patience.

Kala chakra: At the base of the mouth, this acts as a control system for the flow of energy, helping the "bottleneck" of the throat chakra.

OTHER LOWER MINOR CHAKRAS

Naval chakra: A storage area for anxiety and emotions (the knot in the stomach).

Kidney chakra: Concerned with kidney function, the removal of waste and excess fluid.

Pubic chakra: At the pubic bone, this enables sexual expression.

Coccygeal chakra: Near the root chakra at the tailbone, this is associated with physical energy.

Perineal chakra: At the pelvic floor, this is concerned with internal fire.

THE NADIS

Translated as "flowing water" or "river", the nadis are a network of channels through which life energy (prana) flows, connecting to the chakras and other energy points. By working with the chakras, the nadis are stimulated.

According to traditional Indian medicine and Vedic teachings, there are 72,000 nadis in the body.

The three most important to know about are:

Sushumna nadi: Runs from the base of the spine up to the crown of the head through the centre of the body.

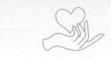

Ida nadi: Runs up the spine to the left of the sushumna nadi, criss-crossing over it at each major chakra like a caduceus, and finishing at the left nostril. It is associated with the right brain (creativity) and yin energy.

Pingala nadi: Runs from the base of the spine at the root chakra upward to the right of the spine, likewise criss-crossing over the sushumna nadi and ida nadi but terminating in the right nostril. It is associated with the left brain (logic) and yang energy.

*"Without knowing energy,
you cannot approach
your soul."*

Ilchi Lee,
Healing Chakras (2010)

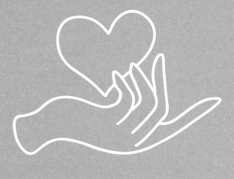

CHAPTER

5

BALANCING
and
UNBLOCKING

Discover meditation, visualization, breathing and yoga techniques for healing, energizing and rebalancing the chakras.

HOW TO UNBLOCK YOUR CHAKRA

You do not need any special equipment –
all you need is quiet time. Some of
the best ways to unblock a chakra
or rebalance an over- or underactive
one include:

1. Breathing practices to encourage
   energy flow

2. Meditations and affirmations to open
   and connect to the chakra

3. Creating alignment in your physical
   body through yoga postures.

"Opening your chakras and allowing cosmic energies to flow through your body will ultimately refresh your spirit and empower your life."

Barbara Marciniak,
Path of Empowerment (2010)

SENSING YOUR CHAKRAS

Some people see colours or images related to each chakra, or feel a warm or tingling sensation in a hand placed over that particular area of the body.

As awareness is a highly individual experience, you will have to experiment to see what works for you. The more you work on it, the better you will be at sensing the energy.

using a pendulum

Hold the pendulum very still a few inches above a chakra point. In a few moments, the pendulum will usually start to move.

A clockwise direction is the healthy rotation of the chakra; if it moves counterclockwise, however, the chakra is spinning out negative energy. Large circles indicate a healthy, robust energy, whereas smaller circles indicate a weak energy.

If the chakra is stagnant, it won't move at all.

feeling it

Try this at home with a friend. Lay your friend on a table or bed and hold your hands a few inches above their body.

Starting from below the groin (the root chakra), move the hands slowly up the central meridian to the top of the head.

You should feel some energy activity, heat or a force field over each chakra point. Note any differences in sensation.

"If you stand beside a person who lies on his back and move the palm of your hand slowly down the midline of his body, about a foot above the skin, you will feel some distinct warm spots. These are the chakras."

Michael Crichton,
Travels (1988)

BREATH RETENTION

This is a simple breathing technique that is great for grounding the root chakra and regulating and calming your breath. Over time you may be able to increase the count from four to eight.

Sit comfortably somewhere quiet and slowly inhale through the nose, counting to four as you breathe in. Hold the breath for a count of four, then slowly exhale through the nose for four. Repeat ten times.

ALTERNATE-NOSTRIL BREATHING

Ida nadi and pingala nadi are associated with the sympathetic (fight or flight) and parasympathetic (rest and digest) nervous systems. This exercise will balance these and promote nadi flow.

1. Sitting in a comfortable position, bring your right hand to your nose and hold the thumb over your right nostril to block it. Take a deep, cleansing breath in and out.

2. Release the thumb and place your index finger over the left nostril, taking a deep cleansing breath in and out.

3. Keep repeating, alternating nostrils, for up to five minutes.

COLOUR CHAKRA BREATHING

Work your way through the chakras to breathe energy into, and open, each one.

You may want to incorporate the mantra for each one, as listed in chapters 1 and 2, or silently repeat an affirmation.

1. Sit comfortably with your legs crossed and your hands lightly resting on your knees, palms down.

   Take a few deep breaths, breathing slowly in through your nose and out through your mouth.

2. Starting with the root chakra, visualize a red vortex or orb of light at the base of the spine and imagine energy flowing through it and pulsating with it. Inhale to direct energy to the chakra, and exhale to allow the energy to settle in place.

3. When you are ready, move on to the orange sacral chakra at the lower abdomen, then the yellow solar plexus at the upper abdomen.

4. Follow with the remaining chakras, working your way up through the pink heart chakra, the turquoise throat chakra, the indigo third eye and finally the violet crown, visualizing each corresponding colour and imagining energy flowing through it.

5. You may feel a little lightheaded or tingly as you finish, so rest quietly and take a few deep breaths. Any tension should now be replaced by feelings of calm and peace.

"Whenever you feel threatened or afraid, you should place your hands over your third chakra, right in the middle of your stomach, and breathe very deliberately and slowly until you feel calm. In doing so you will actually begin to feel stronger and more protected. Breath gives us life and it is the source of our power."

Sonia Choquette,
True Balance (2010)

LION'S BREATH

This exercise is excellent for the throat chakra. Use it before you give a speech or talk or before a conversation, especially if it is on a subject you may find difficult to discuss.

Sit on all fours (tabletop) position, spreading your fingers out wide.

Deeply inhale through your nose. On the exhale, extend your tongue, open your eyes wide, and roar loudly.

PANTING BREATH

Also known as *kapalabhati*, this is a purifying technique that tones the abdominal muscles and directs breath to the solar plexus chakra.

Take a deep inhalation through the nose, expanding the belly out, and then follow with a sequence of short and forceful exhalations through the mouth. With each breath out, the lower belly quickly draws back in towards the spine.

HEART CHAKRAS BREATH

This simple exercise will help you connect to the heart chakra; it is particularly good for promoting self-love.

1. Sitting comfortably in a quiet place, begin breathing deep belly breaths in and out. Notice your belly rise and fall with each expansive breath in and fully empty the lungs on each breath out.

2. Rest your hand on your heart, connect to your heartbeat and feel the rising warmth and love. Imagine your hand cradling the heart as you inhale and exhale, and visualize the heart growing and expanding. Keep breathing for at least ten breaths.

3. When you remove your hand, you should feel a surge of energy in your heart chakra.

EARTH STAR GROUNDING

This visualization can be used for balancing the root chakra, but for a more intense practice, connect to the earth star (see page 100) to foster a wellspring of health and abundance from Mother Earth herself.

1. Stand barefoot on the ground, preferably outside in a garden or park, or at a water's edge or beach. Centre and quieten yourself with a few deep breaths.

2. Now visualize a silver light emerging from the magnetic core of the earth and flowing upwards in through the bottom of your feet and along the spine. Feel the light moving into each chakra and connecting them one by one to the universal (or crown) chakra.

3. Feel the light from above your head moving downward through you into the earth's core in a two-way connection. Visualize the light of the earth star glowing beneath your feet, spreading its healing, restorative natural energy.

variation: Work from the root chakra down to the earth star to draw deep energetic vibrations from the earth and also to discharge excess energy into it.

CHAKRA AFFIRMATIONS

A useful strategy to promote confidence and belief in your abilities, affirmations are simple statements that can help to rebalance underactive or blocked chakras. Repeat them every morning, or use them in combination with meditations, visualizations or other energy work.

root chakra

"I am grounded and rooted like the strong, powerful oak tree."

"I am stable and secure in every way."

"The universe will always provide for me."

sacral chakra

"I flow with passion, inspiration and creativity."

"I freely express my emotions in a balanced and healthy way."

"I embrace pleasure and abundance."

solar plexus chakra

"I am confident, motivated and aligned with my purpose."

"I have the strength and courage to handle any challenge."

"I hold the keys to my own happiness."

heart chakra

"I love and appreciate myself as I am."

"My heart is open to give and receive love."

"I feel gratitude and empathy for others and the world."

throat chakra

"I speak my truth and I allow my voice to be heard."

"I know my authentic self and am unafraid to show it."

"I speak calmly with clarity and confidence and I listen to others."

third eye chakra

"I trust my intuition, perception and wisdom."

"I seek to understand and learn from my life experiences."

"Every day I nurture and grow my spiritual self."

crown chakra

"I am connected to the divine and universal."

*"Everything is connected and I am an
        important part of the whole."*

"I am aligned with my highest self."

"The body is the vehicle, consciousness the driver. Yoga is the path and the chakras are the map."

Anodea Judith,
Chakra Yoga (2015)

YOGA POSES

Yoga offers a great opportunity to release unwanted energy by ushering in life-giving positive energy through breathing techniques and repetitive body postures.

easy pose

A foundation pose that is conducive
to dropping into a meditative state,
this is great for any grounding work to
connect with your root chakra.

1. Simply sit cross-legged on your mat,
   bringing your shins close to your
   torso and tucking each foot under
   the opposite knee.

2. Relax your feet, keep your pelvis
   neutral and place your hands on
   your knees, palms down.

3. Lengthen your tailbone to the floor
   and bring your shoulder blades
   down and back.

ROOT CHACKRA TREE POSE

Standing and balancing poses are great for strengthening the root chakra, the body's foundation. Try this tree pose or just stand in Mountain, the first step, breathing for five to ten deep breaths.

1. Stand upright with your feet facing forward, parallel to each other. Your hips, knees and ankles should stack over one another. This is Mountain pose.

2. Slowly lift your left foot off the ground and turn the sole of the foot to rest on your inner right leg. Press down to the earth through all four corners of your right foot.

3. Slide your left foot upwards, above the knee if possible.

4. Bring your hands together and press the palms together in a prayer position and hold for five deep breaths. Repeat on the other side.

also try: Sitting or Standing Forward Fold, or Warrior II.

SACRAL CHAKRA PIGEON POSE

Hip-openers will strengthen your pelvic floor, where the sacral chakra resides. If you are a woman, try to squeeze and lift the pelvic floor (Kegel exercises) while you are holding the pose.

1. Begin on all-fours (tabletop position). Place your right knee behind your right wrist.

2. Lay your right shin on the floor and slowly inch your right foot forward – your right ankle will be somewhere in front of your left knee.

3. Lengthen your left leg behind you with the top of the foot on the floor and the heel pointing toward the sky.

4. If your hips don't touch the floor, use a yoga block or pillow to support them and keep them level.

5. Extend the spine. Rest your hands on the floor or a yoga block.

6. Hold for five breathes. Repeat on the other side.

also try: Lizard or Chair poses.

SOLAR PLEXUS BOAT POSE

To ignite inner fire and balance the solar plexus, practise the Boat pose.

1. Sit on the floor with your legs bent in front of you and your hands on the mat at your hips.

2. Lean back on your sitting bones and tailbone, engage your core muscles and raise your legs into the air to form a V shape.

3. Extend your arms in front so they're parallel to the floor.

4. Hold for five breaths and repeat two to three times.

also try: Triangle or Reverse Plank poses.

HEART CHAKRA UPWARD DOG POSE

With a fuller lift than that of a Cobra, this pose will open out the heart and help you connect more deeply with yourself and others.

1. Lie on your stomach, with your hands next to the ribs, fingers pointing forward, elbows tucked into the sides.

2. Press the tops of the feet into your mat.

3. On an inhalation, straighten your arms, lifting your chest, hips and legs off the floor.

4. Drop the shoulder blades back, open the chest and hold for up to five breaths.

5. To release, exhale and slowly lower to the floor.

also try: Cobra, Bow or Bridge poses.

THROAT CHAKRA FISH POSE

This pose will open up the throat, reduce anxiety, promote respiration and speaking.

Caution: Do not try this if you have a history of neck problems.

1. Lie flat on your back with arms by the side and palms flat on the mat.

2. Lift the upper body off the ground, bending the elbows, and tip your head back to rest the crown on the mat.

3. Rest your weight on your hips and forearms, keeping the lower body flat on the mat and your throat open to the sky.

4. Breathe deeply in and out through the nose for five breaths, then gently release.

also try: Cat–Cow or Camel pose.

THIRD EYE WIDE-LEGGED FORWARD FOLD

Good for connecting your upper body with your lower by getting the hips above the head and heart to flush the pituitary and pineal glands.

1. Stand in Mountain pose (see page 156), then step your feet hip-width apart, feet facing forward with hands on hips.

2. Lengthen your spine and open your chest on the inhale; on the exhale, fold

forward from the hips to midway point so your back is parallel to the floor.

3. Place your hands underneath your shoulders onto the floor.

4. If you can go further, walk your hands back to hold your ankles and drop your head to a full forward bend.

5. Hold for five breaths.

6. To release, walk yourself back and straighten on an inhale. Return to Mountain pose.

also try: Extended Child's pose, Puppy pose, Dolphin or Humble Warrior.

CROWN CHAKRA RABBIT STAND

This pose is much easier than a headstand for activating the crown chakra and thus stimulating the mind and new ideas.

1. Start in Child's pose by sitting on your heels, spreading your knees hip-width apart and touching your toes together. On an exhale, bend forward to place your torso between your thighs and your forehead resting lightly on the floor.

2. Reach your arms back to hold on to the heels of your feet with your hands.

3. Now inhale and lift the hips up toward the sky and hold for five breaths.

4. To release, lower the hips to the heels and slide back into Child's pose.

also try: Corpse or Crocodile poses.

CHAPTER

6

ENERGY WORK

Crystals, essential oils, massage and other supplemental techniques can be added to your energy work to rebalance the chakras.

root chakra room spray

1 tablespoon vodka

100ml (4 oz) spray bottle

5 drops black pepper essential oil

10 drops frankincense essential oil

10 drops patchouli essential oil

5 drops cedarwood essential oil

Distilled or filtered water

Add the vodka to the spray bottle, then drop in the essential oils. Fill with the distilled water and shake gently. Use as a room spray mist.

protection charms

To protect you and your home from toxic influences, both spiritual and physical, place the root chakra crystals touramaline and jasper near windows or entranceways to your home.

Black touramaline dissipates negativity, while red jasper, considered the blood of Mother Earth by some Native American tribes, enhances physical strength and vitality.

eat orange to rebalance

To help your physical body and energetic body balance in the sacral chakra, choose foods that are in alignment with this chakra: butternut squash, carrots, mango, melon, nuts and seeds, orange citrus, pumpkin, sweet potato.

crystal meditation for vitality

If you are feeling lethargic and lacking in enthusiasm or creativity, your sacral chakra needs firing up! Use carnelian and sunstone crystals with a meditative visualization to increase warmth, energy and sexual vitality.

Lie down in a comfortable position and place the stones over the sacral chakra. Take a few deep breaths, set your intention and visualize a warm orange glow filling the chakra.

Rest for 15 minutes.

personal power tea

This tea blend works to balance the solar plexus, helping strengthen your willpower, stamina and sense of self.

2 teaspoons dried chamomile flowers

1 teaspoon grated fresh ginger root

2 slices fresh lemon

Honey to taste

Place the first three ingredients in a teapot and pour over 250 ml (8 oz) of boiling water. Allow to steep for 5–10 minutes and then strain into a teacup and sweeten with a little honey.

uplifting massage blend

Great for a gentle tummy area massage, this oil will activate the solar plexus chakra, help digestion, detoxify and lift the mood.

10 drops eucalyptus essential oil

10 drops lemongrass essential oil

20 drops rosemary essential oil

100 ml (4 oz) fractionated coconut oil

Add the essential oils to the coconut oil and decant into a glass bottle.

Shake well to combine. To use, warm about a tablespoon in the hands before gently massaging the tummy in a clockwise direction.

manifesting love

An unbalanced heart chakra can result from a romantic break-up, grief or feelings of loneliness and isolation.

Rose quartz is one of the best crystals to help heal a broken heart, promote self-love or bring love back into your life.

Hold rose quartz stones in the hands or over your heart chakra during meditation, or combine with green aventurine, which encourages healing and forgiveness.

*"Do not feel lonely,
the entire universe is
inside you."*

Rumi

"How people treat you is their karma; how you react is yours."

Wayne Dyer

heart healing ritual

For this ritual, you simply need a pen and paper.

First write a letter to someone from your past or to your younger self. Say all the things you wish you'd said and say "goodbye" to that person, or the person you were. Sign it off with love for them.

Then write a "hello" welcome letter to the love you want to invite into your life, or the person you want to become in the future. List all the attributes and desires you want for that person.

Sign off with love and intention.

"*The chakra is a doorway. These are doorways that lead you into other dimensions. But you have to focus on them to the exclusion of everything else.*"

Frederick Lenz,
The Enlightenment Cycle (2002)

mint tea

This tea blend works to balance the throat chakra, helping you speak honestly, communicate your message to the world and open your ears to others.

1 teaspoon dried peppermint leaves

1 teaspoon dried sage leaves

Place the leaves in a teapot and pour over 250 ml (8 oz) of boiling water. Allow to steep for 5–10 minutes and then strain into a teacup.

Sip slowly.

geranium massage

Open up your throat chakra with a neck and shoulder massage using geranium essential oil to relieve stagnation and tension and increase the flow of energy from the lower chakras to the higher.

If you can't get to a trained therapist, try the neck roll at home. Sitting on the floor or a chair, drop your right ear to your right shoulder, then return to centre. Drop your left ear to your left shoulder and return to centre.

Slowly and gradually, and after your muscles are warmed up, work up to full neck-circle rotations.

throat chakra mantra

Humming, chanting, singing and spoken affirmations work well to rebalance and invigorate the throat chakra.

For an easy mantra to release fears, especially when feeling unable to speak up for yourself, simply sit quietly, breathe deeply and repeat the sound "Ham" on the exhale to open your throat channel and free your vocal cords.

throat chakra crystal work

Here are crystals to use for specific throat-chakra-related issues – carry them, place them in crystal grids or wear them in necklaces close to the throat area.

speaking out: Amazonite, the "stone of truth", will help you express yourself clearly.

social anxiety: Larimar will calm nervous energy and alleviate panic and fear.

thoughtfulness: Aquamarine will help with "foot in the mouth" problems and allow to you speak with more care.

angry words: Hemimorphite will pave the way for a peaceful dialogue.

listening:: Angelite will help perception and enable you to hear others' points of view.

connect with the dream world

Blue kyanite will strengthen your third eye chakra.

Place the crystal under your pillow before you go to sleep to enhance dream recall and interpretation, enable lucid dreaming and stimulate your waking-life psychic abilities.

To offer protection and transformation while you sleep, use labradorite.

stargazing ritual

To transcend the cynicism, worldly concerns and "hamster on a wheel" thinking of a blocked third eye chakra, spend a clear night gazing at the stars in the indigo sky to open the mind and gain a new perspective.

If you can't get outside, try meditating on the third eye while focusing on the flame of a candle.

violet light

If you are obsessing about the past or future, and not leading your best life in the present moment, try this crown chakra visualization to bring you to the state of "being".

1. Sit comfortably on a chair with your back straight and your legs and arms uncrossed. Rest your hands on your lap, palms facing up.

2. Close your eyes and find stillness, breathing deeply, and visualize a violet thousand-petalled lotus flower at your crown chakra, opening and pulsating with light.

3. Feel that light dissolving the threads tying you to your past and future, dissolving all blockages and spiralling down into you through the crown chakra.

4. Sit with this channel of violet light emanating through you and allow yourself to be one with the sacred universe. Feel that there is no past or present; there is only now.

5. When you are ready, take a few deep breaths and open your eyes.

"Chakras are organizational centres for the reception, assimilation and transmission of life-force energy. They are the stepping stones between heaven and earth."

Anodea Judith,
Creating on Purpose (2012)